Unlocking the Mystery of Borderline Personality Disorder:

A Survival Guide to Living and Coping with BPD for You and Your Loved Ones

Alison Malkovich

&

Thomas Cox

Additionally, the information in the following pages is intended only for informational purposes and should thus be thought of as universal. As befitting its nature, it is presented without assurance regarding its prolonged validity or interim quality. Trademarks that are mentioned are done without written consent and can in no way be considered an endorsement from the trademark holder.

Table of Contents

Introduction 5

Chapter 1: More Than a Matter of Personality: What is
Borderline Personality Disorder? 7

Chapter 2: The Intersection of Biology and Unhealed
Wounds: Causes of BPD 21

Chapter 3: Treatments: Getting a Diagnosis, Self-
Awareness, Counselling, DBT, and Medication 34

Chapter 4: Tap Into Your Power: How Those with BPD Can
Identify Triggers and Learn New Behaviors......................45

Chapter 5: When Your Loved One Has BPD: The Road to
Acceptance and Healing...53

Chapter 6: Day-to-Day Techniques for Self-Improvement.... 64

Conclusion...78

Introduction

Congratulations on downloading *Unlocking the Mystery of Borderline Personality Disorder: A Survival Guide to Living and Coping with BPD for You and Your Loved Ones.*

The following chapters will discuss Borderline Personality Disorder (also known as BPD). BPD may be one of the least understood psychological diagnoses of our time. It is a disorder often mistaken for manic depression that unknowingly affects the lives of millions of people.

The line between clinical depression and personality disorder is subtle and even healthcare professionals struggle to diagnose their patients accurately. However, the telltale signs of living with BPD, or being in a relationship with someone with BPD, have a visceral truth for those affected. If the information presented rings true for you, then trust your gut. BPD is personal, intense, chaotic, distracting, traumatic, and to its sufferers and those the disorder targets, confusing to the point of despair.

The exciting news is that there is much to be optimistic about modern treatment. The first and most powerful step in identifying and treating the disorder is becoming informed. This book takes that first step with you by compassionately exploring the nine criteria for diagnosis and opening the discussion to make the otherwise chaotic experience of BPD accessible. Origins of the disorder are addressed, as well as the obstacles to a clear professional diagnosis.

Tools and resources are offered, not just for those with BPD, but also for those who are living with a loved one currently suffering from the disorder. One of the most isolating features of BPD is the fact it warps reality. Those who have it cannot connect to the world with constructive, stable relationships and those who are in relationship to someone with BPD are often denied their feelings and truth. The beginning of the road to recovery is learning the truth that you're not alone, you're not crazy, and you're not wrong. By reading this book, you are taking a powerful first step to discovering your truth.

This book does not purport to be a stand-in for a medical professional and you should not approach reading as to diagnosis yourself or a loved one. What is of benefit is a better understanding of this complex disorder that most clinicians struggle to diagnose accurately.

There are plenty of books on this subject on the market, so thanks again for choosing this one! Every effort was made to ensure it is full of as much useful information as possible. If you enjoy this book and find it helpful please leave us a review. Thank you.

Chapter 1:

More Than a Matter of Personality: What is Borderline Personality Disorder?

It is not a simple task to define, assess, or diagnose Borderline Personality Disorder. With most medical diagnoses, one hopes that the underlying concern is easy to spot. With personality disorders, the entire invisible structure of the personality is under review. The clues to its existence lie in relationships: with others, with emotions, with commitments, and primarily, with one's self. It is for this last reason that Borderline is such a hard diagnosis to make. BPD alters a person's ability to relate to their self, to apprehend the reality of their actions and their consequences, as well as engendering a deep feeling of shame. Those who suffer from the disorder are likely to avoid seeking help and treatment because to do so would be to accept that there is an issue at hand. Instead, most borderlines live their lives in denial of any deep, underlying problem at the source of their limitations. However, with those who live with a borderline individual, it is the opposite frustration. Too often, loved ones and close friends live lives in constant doubt of their reality. Is anything *that bad* actually going on with their family member? Are *they* really the crazy one, instead of their friend?

Confusion is one of the telltale experiences of living with or near a Borderline. The amazing evidence is that with a better and deeper understanding of the disorder comes relief.

The fuzziness surrounding the borderline experience is not limited to the personal spheres. In fact, the historical precedent of the disorder includes grey areas and catchall definitions that have led to misconceptions and misunderstandings of the condition to this day. The clinical struggle to capture the essence of BPD reflects the personal confusion and disorientation that those who live with, or close to, the borderline experience. The first step, as with all matters that affect our quality of life, is to gain clarity about the terms of the disorder. Tracking the history of BPD leads to a better understanding of not only what the disorder *is,* but why both clinicians and laypeople can, by no fault of their own, be misled by this shape-shifting and uprooting disorder.

Only in recent years has BPD become a term that enters casual conversations. Celebrities now openly share their borderline diagnoses on Twitter during an age where "He's such a narcissist!" and "What a psychopath!" are half-meant insults thrown around during the day. The definitions around personality disorders are fuzzy. Research into personality disorders is only a recent clinical pursuit of the last century. To aim to understand a personality disorder on a personal level is akin to starting a mythical quest: there is a long, winding road of false starts, monsters, noble guides, victories, and setbacks. At its end, the path to understanding borderline also offers redemption.

While research and the working concept of *borderline syndrome* were ongoing during the late 1950s, BPD did not achieve status as an official diagnosis in the psychiatric manual The Diagnostic and Statistical Manual of Mental Disorders (DSM-III) until 1980. Before this milestone, BPD had first been identified as "borderline syndrome" by psychological researcher Roy Grinker and his team in 1968. This was followed by John Gunderson and Margaret Singer's published research in 1975 that suggested the main identifiable characteristics of the disorder. Gunderson advanced their collaborative work and published a set of metrics that allowed research psychologists to replicate and affirm the validity of BPD. This led to the first DSM definition of 1980, allowing practitioners to now formally assess and diagnose patients with the condition.

However, previous prejudices that the disorder was a "wastebasket" diagnosis have remained prevalent in the field. The fact that BPD takes into account a wide-ranging spectrum of behaviors has left clinicians to view the diagnosis, in certain cases, as a "well, if nothing else fits" last resort. Manic depression, schizophrenia, attention deficit hyperactivity disorder (ADHD), and post-traumatic stress disorder (PTSD) are all formal diagnoses that align with many of BPD's symptoms. While BPD can be co-occurring with many of these conditions, and in fact can exacerbate these conditions, ample studies have shown support for borderline as a distinct condition that deserves its own unique diagnosis and treatment.

The professional confusion surrounding BPD has made the diagnoses somewhat of a cultural taboo. This may be due to the lack of resources or simple solutions to the disorder. There is no one pill to offer borderline as a cure, as with anxiety or depression, and there is no established recovery group, as there is with alcoholism. It is a tricky diagnosis and a recovery that requires multiple levels of care: behavior modification, therapy, psychiatry, soul-searching, and relationship support. What a borderline diagnosis requires the most is time. The road to recovery is often long and hard.

It is unclear in society what to say to someone who shares their borderline diagnosis. However, with ever-increasing research and understanding, this taboo is coming out of the shadows. It is not the nature of the condition that should be left out in the dark but rather its misunderstandings.

Those who have struggled with the condition or have seen it up close will implicitly understand the psychological field's difficulty to get a grip on borderline behavior. The way a sufferer can easily morph from a stable, loving parent into a chaotic victim of a flashback—similar to a post-traumatic episode—and then quickly come out of this chaos only to go on a mad-cleaning spree of the house can easily lead witnesses to believe that there are less complicated and less broad-ranging disorders to diagnose. This is not to imply that bipolar disorder, depression, anxiety, or any other mental health concern is "easier" than borderline, but it is helpful to illuminate how co-occurring disorders can belie one root cause. Just because someone is depressed does not mean they do not have BPD, and just because someone is diagnosed with BPD does not mean they're not depressed. In fact, Borderline Personalities are likely to have these parallel symptoms, but the approach to BPD recovery is quite different from their twin-seeming symptoms.

With a professional field that still has doubts, has only a forty-year history of formally diagnosing its patients as borderline, and the shifting-experience of those with the condition, getting a handle on what BPD *is* can feel like a grey area. Let's look now at the current markers as outlined in the most recent publication of the DSM-IV. The DSM is always under review by a team of experts who continue to pursue evidence-based qualifications for various mental health disorders. Make sure to review the latest DSM publication as this iteration was published in 2013 and will be updated soon. We will then translate what these identifiers may look like into real-life experiences. The following criteria are directly sourced from the DSM-IV (American Psychiatric Association, 2013):

BPD is a pervasive pattern of instability in interpersonal relationships, self-image, and emotion, as well as marked impulsivity beginning by early adulthood and present in a variety of contexts, **as indicated by five (or more)** of the following:

(1) Frantic efforts to avoid real or imagined abandonment

(2) A pattern of unstable and intense interpersonal relationships characterized by extremes between idealization and devaluation (also known as "splitting")

(3) Identity disturbance: Markedly or persistently unstable self-image or sense of self

(4) Impulsive behavior in at least two areas that are potentially self-damaging (e.g., spending, sex, substance abuse, reckless driving, binge eating)

(5) Recurrent suicidal behavior, gestures, or threats, or self-harming behavior

(6) Emotional instability in reaction to day-to-day events (e.g., intense episodic sadness, irritability, or anxiety usually lasting a few hours and only rarely more than a few days)

(7) Chronic feelings of emptiness

(8) Inappropriate, intense anger or difficulty controlling anger (e.g., frequent displays of temper, constant anger, recurrent physical fights)

(9) Transient, stress-related paranoid ideation or severe dissociative symptoms

One of the key insights from the above is the fact that, for each category, a pervasive or on-going pattern of behavior must be true for the borderline individual. An acute episode of intense abandonment stress from a relationship break-up is reasonable; a relationship pattern over a decade of avoiding intimate, stable relationships is not.

Pervasive is meant to be understood as inhibiting satisfactory achievement or advancement towards life goals. For example, a pervasive feeling of emptiness would manifest as chronic feelings of low self-worth. This could show up in the form of missed job opportunities, abusive relationships, poor hygiene, low ambition, distant or infrequent friendships, or long stretches of boredom without relief. "Impulsive behavior in at least two areas that are potentially self-damaging (e.g., spending, sex, substance abuse, reckless driving, binge eating)," may appear on a spectrum. Impulsive spending could look like a maxed out credit card or a non-essential big buy, such as a new car, or it could be frequent splurges on Amazon to the point of never having savings. The key indicator is whether the behavior is interrupting or is harmful to your quality of life. If a goal you have, or one of your family members has, is to own a house but instead, you perpetually plunk money into shopping sprees or nights out, this could be identified as harmful behavior as it is preventing you from achieving a life goal. Keep in mind, five of the nine identifiers must be met concurrently to assess borderline behavior.

Now, those who live close to the borderline experience may see reflections of themselves in the above categories. This is normal. A child of a parent with BPD will grow up within an environment that establishes the above patterns of behavior as norms. A child who is frequently a witness to their parent's suicidal ideations will either consciously or unconsciously come to learn this pattern as normal, or expected, as a reaction to life stressors. A spouse of a partner with BPD may come to expect intense, irrational periods of rage to the point where the spouse believes their actions, whether minor or calculated, are worthy of an inappropriate response.

It is common for those associated closely with the disorder to begin to identify themselves as having borderline tendencies. First, this book is not designed to be a clinical tool and what is outlined here cannot serve as a replacement for proper professional treatment. Even if, after reading the above symptoms, you have a revelation that a loved one's behavior, or your own, fit five or more of the categories, do not take this to be a diagnosis. What is useful is reflecting upon the categories above and starting to see how patterns, yours or others, may have manifested in your life. Steps on obtaining a meaningful diagnosis will be addressed before this chapter's end.

Borderline Personality Disorder is on a spectrum and each case will look unique to each individual. Each category of behavior may express itself to varying degrees and in contrasting directions. Emotional instability in reaction to day-to-day events (e.g., intense episodic sadness, irritability, or anxiety usually lasting a few hours and only rarely more than a few days) may look like an evening of sobbing after watching an emotionally fraught commercial on TV or it may be a swell of anger, slamming doors, or reactionary, hate-fueled emails after a verbal conflict with a family member. While the second example seems to have more just cause for reaction, the key concern is the appropriateness and proportion of the reaction.

Categories such as, "Identity disturbance: Markedly or persistently unstable self-image or sense of self," are more difficult to quantify than the more external-facing categories of impulsive behavior and unstable relationships. What is good to remember is that these categories lead to the patterns that can be observed. If these categories ring true to you upon first glance, then trust your gut. However, as you read further and learn more about the origins of borderline in the next chapter, the reasons for these patterns will become clearer.

No matter the unique pattern of behavior for the borderline, whether it is five or all nine of the identified categories, what becomes apparent is the shift in reality for both the sufferer and those in a relationship with the borderline. A partner of a borderline personality may slip into a push-pull dynamic with someone who is persistently subject to the "extremes between idealization and devaluation (also known as "splitting")." This push-pull between polar opposite treatments may be internalized as the fault of the partner, which may lead them to begin to devalue their selves until the idealization-phase comes back on. The borderline behavior operates within its own sphere of convincing logic. It can feel a bit like a cruel magic trick when a family member loves you one day, despises you the next, and then makes you a cup of tea with a hug on the third. Reality becomes disordered and a sense of self and truth is distorted for all parties involved.

The main objective of all the symptoms serving a borderline personality is to avoid abandonment. This is why patterns of behavior will be specific to each individual and situation. For example, "Frantic efforts to avoid real or imagined abandonment," can be clearly seen in circumstances where the abandonment is imagined. Rites of passage and life milestones are ripe events for borderlines to become triggered. A son or daughter marrying and "leaving" the family may incite a borderline parent to threaten to never speak to their child again as a desperate attempt to avoid accepting that they are no longer a child. A husband who accepts a job that travels out-of-town a few times a month may be met by a borderline wife with infidelity. This would be an inappropriate and frantic response to incite jealousy or retribution for her perceived "abandonment." Even in the difficult, yet normal, event of

14

experiencing a death in the family may be perceived by the borderline individual as an abandonment and set off a physical or emotional tantrum that is inappropriate for their grief.

Those living within this dynamic can feel blindsided, confused, frustrated, helpless, guilty, ashamed, angry, and may dissociate (or emotionally) detach from their immediate environment. BPD does not exist in a vacuum in this way. While more traditional disorders such as depression, anxiety, and even bipolar disorder will certainly create discord within close relationships, Borderline Personality Disorder will go after those relationships specifically as its target. It can be painful, disruptive, and, in its worst case, completely destructive.

Should you be dealing currently with what you may suspect to be borderline behavior or your own condition, remember: there is help and relief.

The first step is to find a mental health professional. There are professional healthcare practitioners who are trained to treat BPD. This is important to ask when first approaching a therapist or psychiatrist. If you are currently working with a mental health counselor or clinician, it is appropriate to ask if they are trained in assessing and treating BPD, and if not, if they know of local physicians or therapists who do. If you only have access to a GP (General Physician or Family Doctor), ask them if they can recommend a therapist or psychiatrist. This can be daunting for some, but remember, all healthcare professionals are there to help *you,* and you should not feel the slightest bit of guilt or embarrassment if you need to find a better fit for your needs.

Know that if you come across any resistance from a psychiatrist who waves a hand in the face of considering borderline personality concerns, then this is a red flag that they are possibly not the strongest support system for you or your loved one. It is rare, but within the medical field, there can be resistance to changing treatments or lines of thinking due to outdated beliefs. The appropriate response from your practitioner is always one of support, curiosity to your concerns, and an explanation of their course of reasoning. You are entitled to respect on your healthcare journey.

Getting a meaningful diagnosis can often be a path of trial and error. It is not uncommon for a BPD individual to receive a diagnosis for either an overlapping, co-occurring, or incorrect disorder, which still provides some relief. Remember that any step towards health is a good step. While the idea of achieving a BPD diagnosis for a resistant family member may feel overwhelming, and may eventually prove too much for that family member to accept, any steps towards clarity, enlightenment, and help are enormous and should be celebrated.

If you feel you are exhibiting borderline tendencies and are met with other recommendations (EMDR: Eye Movement Desensitization and Reprocessing is a common treatment for those suffering from PTSD), do not feel rushed into an official diagnosis. Take each step of your healing with awareness and note what helps and what does not. Borderline is a disorder that is expressed over decades and most likely took years in childhood to develop. There is no quick fix or overnight recovery.

It is helpful to set your mind as a patient would after a severe car accident where they lost their ability to walk. Learning to walk again takes time and will be frustrating. It is doubly frustrating to have to relearn a skill that should be in place after childhood. Yet, life is full of obstacles and it is well worth the effort to give yourself a second chance at a healthy, stable life. Recovery from borderline will take time, but progress will be made with each effort to recover.

If you return no leads after inquiring to therapists and psychiatrists if they experienced with BPD, you can also contact your health insurance and ask for a list of practitioners with BPD experience under your plan. If you do not have insurance, you may qualify for free or subsidized support from your state or province department of mental health and/or social services. Universities are often a source of low-cost, quality health care, as their graduate and doctoral students offer sliding scales or reduced fee treatment in exchange for experience. The most important detail is to find help that is well versed in personality disorder issues. You do not need to be an expert, but one of the most pivotal people in your support network should be.

A large portion of treatment will be self-help activities and exercises. A good way to start down this path is exactly what you're doing now: becoming informed. At the end of this book, there will be a list of recommended further reading. Remain curious and compliment yourself for being an engaged participant in your mental health. You'll be better able to find a mental health practitioner to meet your needs the more you become aware of what rings true for you. The truth is clarifying. Let this be your guide.

Once you have made either your first appointment or an appointment specifically to address your BPD concerns, then it may be helpful to know what will happen next. Your therapist or psychiatrist will proceed with an assessment that may take several forms and have, or not have, several components. First, your doctor or counselor may ask you to answer a series of personal questions, much like an interview, to start developing a pattern of overall behavior. Be as honest and clear as you can in your answers and do not worry if you're "fitting the profile" or not. Try to provide examples as they come to you, or anecdotes that may have caused you concern over the years. Remember that your worth as a person, or goodness, is not determined by these answers or diagnosis. They are just questions and accounts of behavior. Behavior is learned, and with great effort, can be changed.

You may also be instructed to fill out a written questionnaire that either mirrors their questions or goes into further details about your life circumstance. Do not worry about being judged or looking "weird." The more honest and accurate your answers, the better help you will be able to receive. A component that may be included in your assessment, only with your permission, is an interview with loved ones or family members to get further insight into how your symptoms are affecting you. If you have concerns with their answers, you should voice these to your doctor. If you feel they may give an inaccurate response, then share this. Do not ultimately be concerned with their answers. The total picture of your symptoms will be rooted in your experience and will be kept confidential with your healthcare professional.

What may come as a relief or further frustration, depending on how you currently feel about your situation, is a diagnosis may not come quickly. Some healthcare professionals prefer to work with clients for at least a year or more before diagnosing a patient as borderline. This is okay, yet understandably frustrating. Often, all we want is an answer to what has been causing us so much pain. However, the good news is that treatment does not begin with a diagnosis.

The pattern of inappropriate behaviors, unstable relationships, and unhealthy relationship to self will all be elements of treatment and discussion well before a borderline diagnosis.

This is true whether you are concerned you have BPD or you are a loved one dealing with the effects of borderline behavior. Finding a trained clinician is the most powerful first step in the borderline journey, and their supportive work can often address issues of resentment, hurt, anger, regret, and dissociation *before and in order to* get a patient to a place where they are ready to work with the deeper themes of borderline life. While it may be tempting to want a one-to-one, problem-to-solution relationship between treatment and disorder, recovering from borderline is a circuitous path, rich with reward, and even periods of seeming regression may offer a key to opening the next door to progress.

The ultimate reckoning for the borderline individual and those who live in their wake is to consider deeply, *"What do I want my relationship to life, and to my loved ones, to be?"* BPD is the interloper to these goals. BPD behavior sets about a destructive, habitual path of removing quality and stability from relationships to others, to life, and to the self.

A borderline individual will not be able to stabilize a sense of self and thus will create a black-and-white worldview where friends are idealized one day and vilified the next. Their worldview will tell them that goals are "now or never" and that people are "*always* hurting them" or "*never* understanding them." There is a false sense of security that borderlines have by controlling others through their behavior. There is never a grey area or a middle ground from their point of view. Either the world is *completely* supporting them or *totally* abandoning them. They will go to desperate ends to prevent this perceived abandonment.

Victims of borderline behavior may feel smothered, confused as to their own identity, where they begin and end, and what, if anything, they can do to stop their loved one's pain. What proper treatment will start to reveal is that the self is fluid and flexible, designed to meet different needs at different hours, and does not have to be a slave to the false notion that everyone is going to leave you. It is a heroic work to dive into the root causes of borderline behavior. In the next chapter, we will look at the source of this disorder that affects nearly 2% of the population, and the countless many that surround its reach. There is hope and you can get better. Many of those with BPD have gone on to live successful, healthy, fulfilling lives.

For those who love someone with borderline tendencies, there is a great hope for your journey as well. Understanding BPD as a condition that is not yours, nor your loved one's fault, is vital. To get to this understanding, there is a necessary reckoning for the trials and pain that you've experienced. There is also healing offered in developing compassion for the origins of BPD. For anyone who has been touched by an experience with BPD, it is safe to say you already have a deep capacity for empathy and the personal tools necessary to get your life back on track. No matter how difficult the journey, know that you are not alone, and there is light at the end of the tunnel.

Chapter 2:

The Intersection of Biology and Unhealed Wounds: Causes of BPD

"Your biography becomes your biology. This biography includes the totality of your choices, the things you feed your body – your thoughts, your actions, your food – the things you feed your life." – Caroline Myss

Due to Borderline Personality Disorder's relatively recent establishment as a clinical condition with its DSM qualification in 1980, the explanation for the how's and why's of this disorder are not without debate. There just has not been enough time for research to point the finger at any one culprit. The evidence-based research that is available on BPD does not conclusively show it to be purely a biochemical condition nor the isolated result of external influences. What is clear, at this point, is that BPD is a dynamic disorder and it is highly unlikely that its development is purely due to nature or purely due to nurture.

Genetic susceptibility has been agreed to be a key factor by certain experts. However, when discussing BPD the discussion is about a disordered personality. It may be convenient to think of the complicated mechanisms of personality being rooted within biology. In fact, this premise is what the majority of Western medicine is founded upon. Unfortunately, the expression of an individual's personality, at the time of this writing, has not been pinpointed on the human genome. The susceptibility clinical psychologists and researchers have identified when it comes to BPD are the genetic factors that make a person similarly susceptible to depression and anxiety. It stands to reason, then, to ask, "If a person is biologically susceptible to depression, then what factors determine whether that person falls into the arguably more challenging category of personality disorder?"

This is where we will depart from looking to biology solely for an answer. In fact, as we are dealing with personality, we will look at the psychological components first in order to find a relationship with the disorder's impact on an individual's biochemistry. Personality, just like our bodies, has a distinct structure. Personality, just like our biology, needs specific sources of energy and support in order to grow. Most importantly, our personalities, just as our physical selves, desire and require homeostasis, an equilibrium of its interdependent parts.

It may be difficult to imagine what building blocks there are to a personality. If you were to describe yourself, what would you say? That you're kind, curious, and energetic? That you're serious, aloof, and loyal? Is there a serious-to-silly element to the structure of personality that is turned either on or off? Does your personality feel inevitable? Do you feel you can change it if you wanted to? Just what exactly is a personality, to begin with?

There is a psychological map to personality development. As with most psychological endeavors, there are various schools of thought about how precise this map is, and where all its coordinates lie. Carl Jung, the preeminent psychologist of the mid-20th century, evolved Freud's work of the id, ego, and superego to develop a theory of personality that expands over a lifetime. Jung focuses on personality as the *psyche*, the totality of a human's consciousness: thoughts, feelings, behavior, and the unconscious. To Jung, personality was an achievement and not an innate experience for an individual. To achieve a successful personality is the work of a *lifetime*. Jung wrote that personality, at its most complete, was:

"The supreme realization of the innate idiosyncrasy of a living being, it is an act of high courage flung in the face of life, the absolute affirmation of all that constitutes the individual, the most successful adaptation to the universal conditions of existence coupled with the greatest possible freedom for self-determination."

The structure of the personality, according to Jung, consisted of an upstairs-downstairs configuration. The upstairs contains the ego, which is conscious of thought, feeling, and behavior. The downstairs is the unconscious. This is the area of the psyche that is filled with archetypal imagery and patterns, impulses, desires, and fears. The ego acts as the security guard between these two realms. If a desire, say an intense longing for a romantic partner, is let upstairs by the ego, then this desire becomes a conscious thought and goal. If left unconscious, the desire may affect the individual's behavior but be left unknown. The goal, so said Jung, is for the ego to achieve a sense of *continuity* and *identity* for an individual's psyche.

Say, for example, Marie, a single woman in her mid-thirties, wants to have a child. If Marie's ego willingly allows her to make this desire known to herself, she is able to act in constructive ways to achieve her goal. If Marie has always known herself to be ambitious, resourceful, smart, and open to change, then there is *continuity* in her psychic realm about herself. "Well, I've always gone with the flow and pursued my interests. Maybe I'll start researching freezing my eggs or adoption if I do not find a partner in the next year." This, despite whatever feelings may arise for Marie, would be a reasonable response.

However, if Marie has always known herself to be ashamed of asking for help, guilty for not meeting societal expectations, and resenting what she does not have, her ego may turn into a bouncer and body-check any conscious recognition about her deeper desire to have a child. She may go to great lengths to keep this realization out-of-mind. Instead of finding a constructive path towards her goals, she may take out her frustrations on others, on herself, or find ways to "tune out" the noise. The problem lies in the fact that, just as it is a law of physics for energy to never be destroyed only transformed, psychic energy also will not just disappear on demand.

It is this delicate dance of the self that is an expression of personality. Personality is the relationship we have with ourselves as much as with the outside world. When the construction of a healthy personality is interrupted or, at worst case, prohibited, then a disorder in personality may result.

A Wrong Turn In Order To Survive

No matter the psychological map under consideration, the most important outcome in personality development is for a person to be able to accurately relate to and interpret the world around them. Psychologists define a healthy personality as one that has *flexibility*. No, not a personality that can do yoga. Flexibility in personality means that reactions match external circumstances. Say that you were in a classroom and an intense smell of smoke started to waft into the room. Soon after, a fire alarm starting sounding. You may pop up from your desk, shout at others to get out quickly, and hurry your way towards the exit. This would be appropriate. Now imagine this response should you be in a grocery store and you happen to drop a can of peaches. It makes a loud noise, but instead of proceeding to the store clerk for help, you jump up, shout at others, and run towards the exit. This may read as comical because the reaction does not fit the size of the event.

People with personality disorders have disproportionate reactions to the events around them. A daughter calls her father who has BPD. She hears him pick up the phone and says, "Hi Dad, how are you? I wanted to call because, I'm so sorry, but I can't come over today like I said I would." Her father switches in a moment from sounding pleasant to erupting, "How dare you! You NEVER do what you say you're going to do!" While he may be disappointed, and it would not be unreasonable to express that disappointment, the turn-on-a-dime dynamic highlights how, from his perspective, what a small slight registers as a fire alarm within him.

Bringing awareness to how you experience your reality is a meditative and useful exercise. Take a moment to explore this now to understand the underlying foundation of a personality disorder better. Think for a moment and imagine a mirror. If you were to hold this mirror up to the room you are sitting in, what would it reflect back? Hopefully, you would have impressions of a calm, inviting space, or perhaps you're reading this in a more hectic location, and then your impressions would adjust to fit. Now, imagine holding up your mirror to a close friend. What do you notice about them? Not just their physical attributes, but how do they make you feel? Hopefully, this too is a list of pleasant, warm feelings. If there is frustration or complicated feelings about this friend, on a scale of 1 to 10, how angry are you with them? How disappointed? Can you sit with yourself and this feeling at the same time? Meaning, if you feel any anger or hurt, can you also recognize there are other feelings to be felt, and that this will pass?

Now, imagine that, while you were quite little you suffered a great loss. Maybe this *did* happen to you. Do not explore the feeling of the event but just recognize how profound losing a parent, a sibling, or a beloved family pet can be at a young age. This event would, understandably, adjust your mirror's reflection to current events. Now, whenever you see another dog in life, your mental-mirror would reflect back the impression of your kind, playful puppy and you would be affected by these recollections. This fondness of memory, or even bittersweet sadness, is appropriate and a part of life.

For those with personality disorders, their mirrors were affected in such a way early on in childhood that, when they attempt to hold a mirror up to their relationships as an adult, they are not conscious of the fact that their mirror is not only incorrect but also badly warped. It is so warped it is distorting everything into a threat. Further, they do not even feel like they are holding the mirror. They feel they are the warped mirror. For the borderline individual, it is very difficult to separate reality from who they feel they are. In a room where it is tense, like a hospital waiting area, a BPD individual may be unable to remain calm and centered. They may feel paranoid and lost, or guilty and ashamed when they are just waiting patiently with everyone else.

The causes for this warping of the mental-mirror have been debated by psychological researchers. Evidence supports that severe incidents of sexual abuse, physical abuse, or emotional abuse can warp the mirror. Amazingly, there are millions of individuals who grow up in face of these traumas who do not become borderline personalities. The reality is that it is not a one-for-one cause and effect. The behavior precipitated by living within this warped-view of the world is readily identified as destructive, but should also be recognized as adaptive. If it were not for this warped-view, the personality would be able to develop clearly. What is important to understand regarding the birth of BPD is that there was a severe interruption for the individual to reflect the world clearly.

Past Trauma as Present Reality

The seeds of personality disorders are planted during childhood trauma. No matter the abuse or event that interrupted the healthy development of personality, the matter at hand is this experience of trauma. BPD typically share a history of early trauma, although the details of which will vary by degree and category. You may only be familiar with the word from hearing about Post-Traumatic Stress Disorder (PTSD), which also was not registered as an official diagnosis until 1980. Trauma as a psychological term may carry severe connotations for you and make it easy to think, "Trauma isn't something that has happened to me" or "that's something only experienced in war or physically violent environments." It can take some personal work to recognize that trauma is a very common experience in life and that a traumatic event can happen in the most otherwise mundane circumstances.

Raphael, now in his 30s, a gifted writer, took a playwriting course in his first year at university. The professor was beloved among the students and her respect was coveted. Raphael worked harder on his scripts than he did for any other course and made the additional effort of work-shopping his pieces outside of class with friends to better his writing. The professor, at the end of year review, told Raphael bluntly that his work was second-rate and to find a different interest to pursue. The next ten years left him in writer's block until he recognized how powerful his professor's words had been on his efforts.

The previous example was traumatic. While it involved no blood or even romantic violation, it was an event that negatively impacted Raphael's behavior and blocked his unconscious desires to be a creative writer. Any event that obstructs who you are as a person is a traumatic event. It is clear when a car crash takes a life, but less clear when an interpersonal interaction takes a part of a personality.

This is why the range of traumatic childhood experiences can vary when considering personality disorders. It could be as clear as persistent physical abuse from a father, or it can be as subtle as the silent neglect from a mother whenever the child is upset. It could be the death of a parent that is never spoken about in an honest way, but rather left as a never-to-be-discussed family secret. It could be an alcoholic sibling whose pervasive lies to a younger sibling shift that child's sense of truth and trust. It could be anything that interrupts a child's sense of reality, self, security, or validation. Anything under this umbrella should rightfully be labeled as traumatic and dealt with as trauma.

Other biographical histories of bullying, neglect, or loss could be within a BPD's profile. It could be the uncertainty of a childhood in foster care. It could be the confusion of growing up in two households where one parent is attentive and loving and the other is neglectful and self-involved. It could be an older sibling who always told you that you would never amount to anything. The traumatic event or events—while useful to know personally and to share with a healthcare professional in order to begin treatment—is less important specifically to understanding the origin of BPD.

The grand theme of the trauma is of transgression and abandonment. Transgression is invading a person's sense of self and privacy, compromising their safety, confusing their sense of selfhood or security, or inflicting abuse. Abandonment is either outright absence (a parent who never comes home on the weekends due to an over-taxing work schedule) or absence of presence (a parent who is always home but is mentally and emotionally absent due to drug use). Transgression and abandonment are two breeds of trauma that directly target who a child is as a person. They are both messages that the child's independence is not worthy of respect, value, or care. The child's birthright of joy, emotional freedom, and self-esteem are sacrificed by the traumatic specters of abandonment and transgressions. The message from the neglectful or transgressed parent to their child is "who you are is not as important as what I need." That child then grows confused about what they need, who they are, if their feelings are appropriate, and if they can trust the person they love not to hurt them. These *fundamental* building blocks of personality are compromised. This is the breeding ground for personality disorders.

Trauma, as a medical term, is defined as an injury of such severity that immediate attention is needed. It is urgent. The invisible trauma in our personal lives to the self and to the psyche, while urgent, typically becomes buried. This is often a matter of survival. If, as a victim of abuse, you found yourself not addressing the real hurt, anger, sadness, or pain of that event until years or even decades later, this speaks to the power of your inner resilience. Often, victims of trauma have to compartmentalize their honest reactions until they are in a safer or more stable environment. Especially children of traumatic incidents will most likely not have the resources or ability to process trauma. Even worse, if the child's caretaker is the abuser, then the child must survive by forgoing her experience of trauma to just live. In the psychological realm, psychic trauma can often take years before attention can be paid.

Growing up in a borderline-inducing environment will demand that this trauma never be addressed. Adults who have BPD or grew up with a borderline loved one will recognize this truth. Asking a borderline parent, "Why do you never let me live my life? It feels like you can never let me go," will be met with a panic, a rage, or some ill-fitting reaction.

Unprocessed trauma is the source of a disordered personality. The BPD never grew up with a personality structure that would allow for a flexible relationship between reality and inner life. A BPD individual will go through a break-up and not experience it as the end of a romance but as the end of their world. Their response may be suicidal ideation or sending persistent emails in a rage to their ex-partner. It is because unprocessed trauma is keeping the borderline individual from being okay just within himself.

Childhood trauma interrupts the ability of the child to trust their reality, their feelings as correct, and their world as hopeful and good. That child, now an adult, will continue to react to the world as if it will fall apart if they do not hold it together. This is why BPD is an intensely confusing disposition for both its sufferers and their loved ones. The BPD individual is doing the best they can, with what they know, to repeat the boundaries they learned as children. Unfortunately, these boundaries were incorrect and caused them pain. Loved ones of BPD will see how much their partners are hurting, but be unable to help heal this historical trauma. The cycle continues until real, professional intervention can be found.

Trauma, no matter how distant, remains until it is healed. Jung claimed that all experiences are remembered and downloaded into the unconscious. Nothing is ever lost. If there is a trauma from when you were six-months-old, before you remember having your first thought, it is still, allegedly, deep within. This may sound frightening or like a fairy-tale prophecy, but the reality is that our pasts build our personalities of today. The aim is for a healthy, integrated, flexible sense of self that can adapt to situations as needed. Unprocessed trauma can derail this development in personality. The borderline individual is trapped within an old reality, full of threats to his existence, and is fighting situations in the present as if they were threats from the past.

Who Does BPD Effect?

Early in awareness for BPD, it was assumed the root cause was mainly sexual abuse experienced as a child. For this reason, there was a significant majority of women diagnosed with BPD over men, as it is a more highly reported trauma for girls than boys. It was also posited that women have a higher diagnosed rate for BPD due to the socialization of women to deny and to invalidate their feelings. This remains speculative. It can also be contested that men are often raised to never seek help for apparent emotional "weakness" and that this is a reason reports for borderline women are higher. These notes on the gender disparity of BPD diagnosis point out how much of the disorder is influenced by societal norms and how the individual, male or female, relates to the outside world.

That said, it is most likely, based on research, that the borderline individual experienced a period of extended abuse rather than one acute event. A one-time horrific event of losing a close friend in a freak accident during childhood is less likely to result in BPD than a prolonged experience of real or threatened abandonment. The formative years of childhood also see the formative years of personality development. The greater the interruption of both by trauma, the more likely the individual is to suffer a disordered personality.

Interestingly, BPD does not express its key characteristics until adolescence or early adulthood. Teenage years, when it is typical to start friendships based on shared personalities and to begin romantic relationships, can be further complicated by BPD. Teens face the additional hurdle of having their experiences and mental health often dismissed as just "the problems of youth" or as "only a phase." Even in adolescence, a healthy individual will be able to establish and maintain close relationships without personal harm or erratic behavior. Do not make the error in believing your feelings are not real, made up, or too intense to be validated. Bringing awareness early to patterns of thought, feeling, and relationships will only benefit you for your entire life.

Young adults often suffer the most from their either diagnosed or undiagnosed BPD. It is at this stage of life that is rife with transition, change, expectation, and social pressure. This is a crucible for those whose personalities have been, unbeknownst to them, altered by biographical or biological trauma. A young adult going off to university, or a recent graduate hunting for a job, or a first relationship moving towards a deeper commitment will all bring out unexamined fears, desires, and coping mechanisms. If the structure of a twenty-two-year old's psyche is not equipped to match the reality of their circumstances with their reactions, then it is safe to say all (inner) hell can break loose.

Young adulthood is also a critical time in personal development, as the habits of personality are not set firmly in stone. Just as a baby bird first learns to fly from its parent and then has to leave the nest and hopefully follow instruction as before, an eighteen-year-old off to university is now being tested on their ability to fly. Will they follow the habits they were raised in? Will they go to bed at the same time every night, eat the same sorts of food that were on their family dinner table, make the same sort of friends, or have the same sorts of interests? More often the case is no. This will be a time of rebellion and experimentation to discover who they *really* are and who they *really* want to be.

The chaotic period of individuation from a family of origin makes it even more difficult to spot what is or is not normal, healthy behavior. The pressing concern when deciding if a disordered personality is in play is the inner experience of the individual. Are there persisting feelings of emptiness? Abandonment? Self-hatred? Are these feelings or reactions to these feelings getting in the way of committed, intimate relationships? Holding jobs? Keeping yourself from harm? These are the concerns that should lead someone to seek help.

Likewise, as the borderline individual matures with age the disorder itself may become less intrusive, even without formal intervention. Studies have observed that BPD does tend to "settle down" with age. The concern remains that triggering events (see Chapter 4) will affect the borderline at the same extreme as the young adult borderline. If one thing is known about life, it is the fact that change is always imminent, and for the fixed, rigid structure of the borderline personality, these changes will be met with resistance and chaos. While BPD can first be assessed in adolescence, and while it may be more prominent in early adulthood, there is no shame or disadvantage to recognizing the condition in later life. In fact, those who have survived with the disorder into their maturity may be better equipped to manage, both personally and financially, the steps necessary to help heal. Regardless of the age or stage in which BPD is identified, it is never too late to heal.

Chapter 3:

Treatments: Getting a Diagnosis, Self-Awareness, Counselling, DBT, and Medication

"The best way out is always through."

— Robert Frost

Start right now with self-awareness. Take a breath. Think about what led you to read this book, right now, today. What feeling did you have before starting it? Breathe again. Notice your hands. What do they feel like? If it is nothing, that's okay. Breathe again. Relax your shoulders. Focus on your neck. How does it feel? Stiff, tight, hot, cold? Simple. Just check in. If you are having trouble noticing how you feel, then just notice that. Think, "I notice it is difficult for me to tell how my neck feels right now, or how I feel in this moment." That's a great start.

The above brief exercise is the smallest but most powerful tool you have to heal and progress with BPD. Self-awareness is not some magical power that only certain people have. Everyone has it. We all have access to self-reflection and we have the ability to sharpen this skill. For those who have BPD or have grown up near it for so long, it may be difficult to engage with yourself on this level. That's okay. Know and trust that it is a process, it will take time, but small steps and seemingly small milestones are, in fact, gigantic leaps forward.

Pursuing treatment for BPD or for its impact on your life is a quest for a happy, safe relationship with yourself. You may have other goals: to fix your family, to secure a loving romantic partnership, to succeed at dreams. The secret is this: these goals are all byproducts of a happy, secure relationship with yourself. You cannot have a happy family life, have a successful marriage, or really experience the realization of your dreams without a rooted sense of self.

Think of your entire being as a glass of water. The water represents all the good things in your life, both real and desired. The water is your family, your friends, your hopes, your dreams, your laughter, your anger, your disappointments, your hopes, and your everything. The glass is *you*. You are holding all these things. You, a glass of water, may take it for granted that you hold such treasures, but every glass does to a certain extent. You are just doing your job as the glass that holds the water. Now, someone with BPD cannot be the glass. They want to be the glass and try so very hard to be like glass, but they are more like a sheet of paper. They curl themselves up into a glass-like posture, but the water bleeds right through. They try to fix things by running around and borrowing glass from others, but this does not work because other people cannot hold your water. They wrestle with the water and yell at it to try to make it stay in a glass-like pose. They just cannot hold the water like a fully formed glass.

The work of therapy and treatment for BPD is the alchemy that will turn a substitute personality, built on the survival mechanism of trauma, into solid, water-carrying glass. It is a reconstructive process. If you have ever experienced talk-therapy or cognitive-behavioral therapy (CBT), the borderline treatment is not like that. Whereas CBT addresses behavior with an aim of improving situations and feelings, treatment for BPD is looking to instruct you on how to rebuild your personality, from the ground up, into a healthy structure. It is a terribly courageous and challenging operation and persistence, compassion, patience, and hard work are necessary.

The same is to be said for those recovering from a loved one's BPD. The aim, however, is not to say you are "wrong" and need "fixing." Borderline Personality Disorder is a diagnosis, not a judgment. The aim is to transform a personal hell into a life-embracing, healthy, flexible spirit. It is a gift to give yourself that second chance which was unfairly denied.

Self-awareness is the first tool in the journey. Take a moment now to breathe. Ask yourself, "Do I want to give myself this gift?"

If you've kept reading to this point, you're on the right track. One of the greatest obstacles to getting treatment is denial on behalf of the BPD individual. The fact that BPD creates a twisted view of reality and the self makes it easy to see how denial could come into play.

Jessica, a woman in her 40s, had been suffering from BPD all her life. Her first marriage ended badly in her late 20s and she had gone through a series of abusive relationships since then. She had always been ambitious in her career but had hit the ceiling, due to the fear that her superiors never really valued her work. Jessica's daughter stopped talking to her after she left for college. Jessica would try to call, but would only get her daughter's voicemail. An email every now and then would let Jessica know that her daughter was okay, but that she was too busy to speak. After seven years of this, Jessica finally was able to press her daughter for an explanation for this avoidance, when all Jessica wanted to let her know was that she loved her: Jessica was "smothering" her. Jessica was gutted. She burst into sobs and felt the sinking feeling she had felt throughout her life: that her daughter, and everyone she ever cared about, would leave her. This one word drove Jessica to the point of wanting to be admitted to the local mental health inpatient center. She was devastated and was unable to stay at home with her intense feelings of hurt and shame. She drove to the clinic but upon parking realized that the only thing her daughter had done was say one word to set her off. When Jessica met with a clinician and discussed her situation, she calmed down and admitted she had been this way before. It was the first time Jessica confessed this reaction was a pattern in her life. "It was a great relief," she wrote, "To let myself finally know something, not someone else, was wrong."

Personal revelations can be cathartic, and it is a testament to how strong a grip BPD can have in a case like Jessica's where so much time is lost because no appropriate intervention is sought or available. This is why there is no replacement for professional help that is informed by training in BPD. Give yourself the best care possible. Do not settle for treatment that does not bring you the relief of an answer and explanation that puts a light where there was once only darkness and confusion.

Dialectical Behavioral Therapy

Dialectical Behavioral Therapy (DBT) is the most commonly used treatment for diagnosed BPD. It is a cognitive therapy and gives patients new skills to deal with difficult emotions and relationship issues. DBT differs from traditional talk-therapy in that there are activities and exercises that are practiced in both private and group settings. Think of it like a gym for your soul where you can strengthen and learn to trust sets of muscles inside your personality you never knew you had.

DBT was developed specifically for the treatment of BPD. The name comes from its emphasis on the dialectical or acting through opposing forces. BPD individuals have great difficulty with holding two opposing truths at the once. The BPD inner-landscape is a series of black-and-white portraits and either-or statements. This relates back to the disorder's origin in childhood where, at some point, an event or person made it very clear it was their life that was important over the child's right to own theirs. DBT is structured to introduce "and" thinking: *I'm angry and you're angry. I'm happy and you're angry, and that's okay. You're right and I'm right, in our own ways.* It is a revolutionary change and thus a powerful modality for treating BPD.

DBT focuses on four main areas of the psyche: **mindfulness**, **emotional regulation**, **interpersonal effectiveness**, and **distress tolerance.**

Mindfulness is the ability to be present in the current moment, as it is. For the borderline individual, being present in the moment is a constant challenge. As their sense of identity is never secure, the borderline will both consciously and unconsciously seek out their next source of substitute identity. For example, if a borderline individual is at work, rather than staying focused on the matter at hand, they may be drifting off in their mind to what their boss is thinking about them right now. They may project, or falsely place their inner-experience onto someone else, and assume their boss thinks they are a slacker. *"I'll prove them!"* the borderline may think and run into their boss' office, seeking positive attention.

The lack of a healthy identity and self-esteem leads the borderline to seek affirmation from others constantly. If not from others, then from status-prizes. If the BPD woman is feeling low about herself, she may run to the store to buy a flattering dress on impulse. Mindfulness is a step toward correcting this compulsive need for outside validation. Practicing mindfulness is practicing being centered in the self and noticing any distractions, or impulses, that flash up and letting these go.

Emotional regulation in DBT means to develop strategies for changing extreme emotions that are causing difficulties in a borderline's life. For example, shame can be a debilitating emotion for a BPD individual. Shame caused by a minor or major incident can send a BPD reeling into either outrage and fury or withdrawal from the world. The work in DBT transforms these experiences into workable events that can be *managed* rather than *suffered*.

There is always a choice when it comes to experiencing emotions. For the BPD individual, this is a radical notion. For some, "just shake it off" or "forget about it" is fine advice. For the borderline, it is a myth. DBT uses tangible, actionable techniques to guide those with BPD or BPD after-effects to a place where they can experience their emotions without being overwhelmed.

Interpersonal effectiveness is the standard for all healthy relationships. Its achievement means being in a relationship with others without black-or-white thinking, all-or-nothing reasoning, nor me-or-you emotional debates. The DBT techniques for interpersonal effectiveness promote a self that is clear about its boundaries in a relationship. Too often, BPD people in relationships feel as if they do not have a right to their own feelings being heard. They were taught by their traumatic experiences to devalue their inner lives for the sake of others. However, this denial of self cannot last. The energetic reality of the inner life will be suppressed until it cannot be contained. This results in outbursts, long-term silent resentments, and the sense of never being understood or accepted as a person.

The limitations of BPD in love are a lack of honest communication. This is not because the BPD individual does not want to be honest, but she truly feels trapped and unable to share her feelings. DBT begins to correct this by practicing assertiveness. This ability to be assertive, not aggressive, engenders a sense of self-respect. The human psyche needs validation from our community. It is necessary for our survival as healthy, functioning members of a society. These skills taught in DBT flourish in both the one-on-one settings as well as the group workshops. It is a courageous voyage to be speaking up for yourself, but the radical experience of stating clearly what you need and then realizing the world does not react as you expect it to is both relieving and life-affirming.

Distress tolerance may be the most direct address to the BPD disposition. Borderline personalities cannot tolerate actual or perceived stress. A manageable trigger for anyone else will register as an acute pain for the borderline. It is almost like having the volume turned up to eleven when everyone else is only hearing a light background noise. The normal reaction of the BPD is to escape from this intolerable pain.

It is this aspect of DBT that practices *radical acceptance.* The therapy respects the hard truth of reality that there will be difficult times. DBT increases the ability of the BPD individual to tolerate negative experiences rather than run away from them. Radical acceptance encourages statements such as, *Yes, this is happening right now and it is very bad and I'm not going to do anything but sit here. I am okay.* The dynamic experience of working with a trained counselor in this regard cannot be matched. It is powerful to sit in a room and increase your capacity for resilience. Imagine if everyone worked as hard on themselves as those who seek healing. It would change the landscape of how often we are kind to each other rather than reactionary.

DBT relies on both group work and one-on-one counseling. Your therapist may agree that you only need one or the other, or both, to support you where you are in your recovery. If you are intimidated by a group setting, please first know that communal healing is a long-standing tradition in many cultures and what may first seem strange or uncommon can provide a depth of understanding and community that you never thought possible. If you are apprehensive about private therapy or have had bad experiences in the past with counseling, please also know this is not uncommon. The best thing you can do is to read forums, articles, and books about other people who shared a similar experience to gain perspective that you are not alone.

Therapy is a profession that exists to help people fully integrate themselves and lives in order to experience joy, satisfaction, and progress. Therapy is also what we offer our friends, family, and loved ones when they are going through a difficult time in their lives. It is not acknowledged as thus, but it is still support with the intent to heal our troubled friends. It is not wrong, or shameful, to need help. Professional therapy is a requirement for the treatment of BPD. However, recognize if you have concerns about starting professional treatment that you have most likely received help or advice from the family before, and it is not so strange to seek comfort and understanding from others. The difference is, while friends and family probably have offered you words and gestures that provided temporary relief, licensed professionals will offer you a path to personal freedom.

Supplementary Care

There is no question that our behavior influences our biology. While in the previous chapter focus was placed on the origin of BPD as unprocessed childhood trauma and its pursuant coping strategies, there is a level of the disorder that rightly affects the body and may require medical or alternative support.

Neuroscientists have shown how positive affirmations can directly affect and improve brain chemistry. If there is evidence for positive affirmations affecting brain chemistry, then it is not too far a leap to suggest that the low self-worth statements and near-constant anxiety BPD can incite will lead to inverse damage.

Regardless of a direct link between BPD and the brain, studies are clear that co-occurring or overlapping health issues arise within the borderline personality. Depression and anxiety are common and a common co-diagnosis or in some cases, false preliminary diagnosis is bipolar disorder. All these mental health concerns are traditionally treated by psychiatrists with medications that interact with neurotransmitters to reshape the map of your brain chemistry.

Medication with any diagnosis that is made by a licensed professional—preferably a practitioner in the mental health field (vs. a family doctor)—can be appropriate and beneficial. Even when treating a bipolar diagnosis that is eventually revealed to be BPD, the relief that mood stabilizers used for bipolar treatment could be a lifesaver. They could offer temporary relief until deeper issues can be addressed. Prescriptions for anxiety and depression could be the best support for your physical and mental health until you are more stable in your intrapersonal treatment.

It is wise to approach supplementary care with the mindset that they are indeed supplements to therapeutic core work. The trial-and-error process of finding the right prescriptions can be a walk in the park for some or a never-ending struggle for others.

Kevin, 25, was able to stabilize his ever-decreasing depressed moods that would last a week to a month with the help of SSRI (Selective Serotonin Reuptake Inhibitors). This allowed him to have the willpower to find an appropriate therapist experienced in DBT. The thought of finding a counselor before starting medication seemed impossible.

Sarah, 37, usually known for her bubbly attitude in her family, struggled with a misdiagnosis of bipolar and a decade of start-stop medications to address her complaints. It wasn't until Sarah began DBT therapy, that she began to get a sense of her best self again. Medication in both cases, one explicitly positive and the other frustrating, served its purpose: to bring patients closer to the work that needs to be done.

It is easy in a Westernized culture where television ads for the latest depression medication or sleep prescription bombard our screens to believe that medication is designed to be *the* answer. Prescription medications are definitely the answer for patients who need mood stabilization after a prolonged imbalance. Those who need relief from overwhelming despair or who need recourse after not finding an answer elsewhere. There is no right or wrong path for anyone while seeking treatment. Even when medical intervention is needed, medication is never the *whole* answer. Always ask your doctor about any concerns you have about medications you are currently taking or are interested in learning more about.

Outside of medication, other modalities can be very beneficial as you pursue recovery either with a BPD diagnosis or before confirmation of a diagnosis. Body and spiritual care practices are an excellent way to relieve stress and increase your sense of self-awareness. Yoga, massages, acupuncture, Reiki, Tai Chi, and meditation are all excellent starts. In fact, any practice that asks you to be still and focus on yourself will increase your inner resilience when faced with a distressing event. These modalities are becoming accessible in Western countries and insurances now offer benefits for alternative care depending on your coverage. If getting to a yoga studio for the first time seems intimidating, or if meditation seems awkward, try searching instructional videos online. It can be very powerful just to observe others practicing a skill that you would like to learn. In an ever-connected world, you are not alone, and that especially applies to BPD individuals seeking a healthier life.

Chapter 4:

Tap Into Your Power: How Those with BPD Can Identify Triggers and Learn New Behaviors

There is an ever-growing list of BPD individuals who are living happy, successful lives full of stable relationships. This speaks to the power of therapy and early intervention that has become more widespread since the 1980s. The spark of insight from learning for the first time just what, exactly, is going on with their inner lives can motivate those with BPD to pursue recovery through its uphill battle. "I thought I would never know what was wrong with me!" Sarah in her early 50s exclaimed after being asked what the positive part of having a BPD diagnosis. "I thought I was crazy! I thought there was nothing to be done and I would just always feel like a failure. Now, I know that it is a disorder that tricks your mind, and I think your spirit, into believing you are a failure. You're not at all."

There are an exuberance and freedom in receiving the correct name for a disease or disorder. "There are two questions we ask in medicine," writes Dr. Robyn Parker, Ph.D., "Is there a name for it and can we do something for it." It also provides patients with a sense of relief that they give their loved ones a clinical explanation for their behavior, rather than a confusing mix of emotions about the negativity they have caused. "It depersonalizes it, which is a relief when the whole bloody thing is so personal," concludes Sarah.

The caveat here is that no one else can prepare you for a diagnosis except yourself. Loved ones might be tempted to push you in a direction you are perhaps uncomfortable with. This may increase acting out and defending your right to seek help when you are ready. However, be advised, if loved ones are trying to reach out to you with concern, it is because they deeply care about you, your relationship, and want to see you well.

A grown adult daughter may drive her BPD parent to the therapist's office twice weekly and that therapist may state repeatedly it is time to address her concern of borderline behavior but this still does not mean that a patient is ready to pursue treatment. Help cannot be forced; it must be received. The optimism that may come with the initial awakening to borderline, and the explanation it holds for otherwise mysterious internal conflict and dead-end relationships, can be enough to open the BPD individual to receiving help. This is the grace of knowledge. Commend yourself for taking the first step towards healing by first educating yourself on options for recovery.

The truth is that BPD individuals have survived personal nightmares and this is a great testament to their strength. If you have experienced a childhood trauma and are standing here today, please know that this shows an enormous capacity for inner-strength, willpower, and the ingenuity to survive desperate circumstances. Trauma has no doubt cost you more than you want to bear. The inner resources necessary to confront, heal, and release these traumas is already self-evident. You are strong because you are a survivor.

It is very possible to apply the techniques of Dialectical Behavioral Therapy to your life and being to progress. This reading cannot serve as a substitute for professional healthcare and any exercises or advice presented here is meant to be an exploration and cannot be considered medical treatment. The following are helpful steps to bring a new dialogue within yourself and fortify your path in recovery. Even if you are doubtful about having a BPD status, or you are certain that you are affected, these exercises can help empower you in both your relationships and life path. Let's begin.

Identifying Triggers

The paradox of identifying BPD within oneself becomes obvious: how can you see yourself clearly when the root issue is that nothing is clear? This is why paying attention to behavior is so important. Just as it would be unfair to ask an infant how they are feeling and expect an articulate, accurate answer, it is almost unfair to expect those with BPD to give an accurate, articulate account of what their emotions are doing during an upset. The feelings are too overpowering and the sense of reality is so warped that any explanation will most likely exponentially add to the distress. What is fair to observe with an upset infant is their behavior. If a baby is crying, then a parent knows there is a series of issues to be addressed: change of diaper, hunger, a hug, a beloved stuffed animal gone missing. The behavior of crying clues the parent in. Later on in the terrible-twos, paying attention to behavior can clue a parent into the real cause of upset beyond the cry-storms of, "I want apple juice!" If the toddler is throwing their fists around and stomping, it may be a sign of exhaustion and how good a nap (and not a juice) would be. In a similar way, borderline individuals must begin to look at their behavior for information about their needs, rather than their overwhelming emotions.

This is not to infantilize BPD individuals or their emotions at all. In fact, it is quite the opposite. Borderline individuals should turn to and treat their inner life with the same loving,

47

patient care a parent would a child. The emotional, reckless inner storms of the borderline personality will not give logical, rational explanations for their existence. Most likely, these storms will come on in a flash, unbeknownst to the BPD individual of their cause, and will overwhelm them to the point of not being able to distinguish a crisis from a non-threatening course of events. If, instead of focusing on the extreme upset or outpouring of anger, the BPD individual notes how they are slamming doors, or screaming into the phone, or pacing relentlessly around the house, then valuable information beings to build. The core transformation that is going to take place is a new pattern of alternative behaviors in the face of similar emotions. The emotions will evolve and lessen over time, but not without a change in behavior first.

"I used to get into the car, slam the door shut, then open it and slam it again. I didn't even notice my daughter was crying," shared recovering BPD parent, Mindy. "Honestly, I didn't know I was slamming the door shut until my daughter grew up and confessed how frightening those episodes were. It was heart-wrenching to hear."

In their heart of hearts, those with BPD do *not* want to be exhibiting the unbridled emotions or behavior that is causing their loved ones, and their own lives, grief. It is, in fact, their deep want to be loved and share the love that has led to a maladaptive set of coping mechanisms that no longer match the size or reality of their situations. Those with the disorder are much like children who are out to play in the backyard but have no authority figure to let them know what it is time to come in. Left unsupervised, the children go off, get lost, become frightened, act out, and demand attention in order to be rescued. The miracle of healing and seeking treatment is that the BPD individual can reclaim their right to personal security and end the madness of being victim to their intense emotional episodes.

Perhaps you feel overwhelmed right now just considering the idea of changing behavior. Please know that no matter how you think or feel, change is possible. A BPD diagnosis brings a lot of hope and many people recover. Recovery looks different for every patient and it also exists within a continuum. What is promised, with dedication and applied compassion from yourself and a licensed clinician, is relief from self-harm, broken relationships, and a life that feels at the whim of any emotion that passes through.

An Emotional Bank Account

Go ahead, take out a notepad or journal, and start to jot down a list. The list is going to be based on three-time intervals: today, last week, and last month. Try to identify any and every moment you were upset in some form. Whether it was anger, irritation, jealousy, sadness, down, depression, or boredom. Set a timer for ten minutes and just write what comes up. If you only get through one or two things, do not worry; this is great. Take ten minutes now and write down your list.

Now, take a step back and see what kind of event started each emotion. Were they all in conflicts with other people? Were they moments when you were alone? Make a note of any themes or connections you see.

Now rank each event on a level of 1 to 5. 1 will represent a level of emotion that was present but did not disrupt your day. 5 represents a level of emotion that was almost intolerable. Score all your events now.

Look at the events that you have ranked the highest. Go ahead and list the details of the incident. Focus on what happened immediately prior to your upset and then detail what behaviors were present during your elevated emotional state. Place no judgments on either what caused your reaction or what happened during your reaction.

The process you just completed is a self-inventory. Self-inventories serve as an emotional bank account. Just like money, emotions are a finite resource that you have a certain store of every day. Just like your financial health, your emotional health depends on taking stock of your resources, making sure nothing is overtaxing your account, and that you are spending your emotions wisely.

Look at your just completed self-inventory. Now, without labeling any event as "wrong," which behaviors or feelings do you feel were perhaps a waste of energy, or emotional value misspent? Which ones do you still feel strongly about and still want to invest energy into? Were there any negative consequences from "overspending" your emotional account during any one day? If so, list these consequences and rank them from 1 to 5 (1 being a minor inconvenience to 5 being a strong regret). Try to determine which kinds of triggering events led to the more costly and severe emotions. Were they difficult interactions with friends? Disappointments from loved ones? The general feeling of being ignored or even bored?

This simple account, which you can repeat daily, or practice once a week, is a very strong tool in starting to record and examine behavior. Keeping a log of triggering events and resultant behavior, without judgment, can be a vital tool to share with your therapist. They say a picture is worth a thousand words and in this case, an emotional ledger is worth your sanity. All joking aside, the process of taking your internal experience and setting it down onto paper then taking it under review and then interpreting its larger themes is nothing short of inviting a miracle to work itself during your recovery. *Behavior will not change without awareness. Awareness will not begin without a practice.* All the power you need is in the simplicity of paying attention to your behavior and cracking the shell on how it is either serving or denying your life.

The more you take an emotional bank account and self-inventory, the more you'll be able to change your behavior. The pace of change may feel glacial. This is normal and it is vital you remain patient with yourself. The key is this: the more you notice a trigger, a reaction, and your feelings about how these two feelings came to pass, the more information you send to your brain in order for it to utilize its neuroplasticity to make changes. Ingrained habits live blissfully in ignorance.

If you wake up every day and immediately hit your snooze button, this behavior will continue indefinitely if you never notice that is precisely what you're doing every day. As soon as you are aware of your snoozing, now you are able to reflect on its existence. *I hit snooze every morning. Is it every morning? Yes, for three days now I've noticed. Will it happen tomorrow?* Remain curious. You are allowed to notice behavior on and on until you are ready to make a decision on what to do about it. *It's been 7 weeks of hitting the snooze alarm, I wonder what it would be like if I didn't.* Should it turn out that you are a happier camper forgoing snooze and an alarm clock altogether, then success!

You discovered what works for you. With BPD behavior, most of the intense mechanisms of the disorder are on autopilot. Going into a rage upon any personal slight for some borderline individuals is akin to automatically hitting the snooze every morning after the alarm. The *only* method of changing behavior is to notice it. Start growing your emotional bank account today. There is no need to have the intention to change anything, to begin with. Just begin with noticing how your day flows and when it is interrupted. Your personal power lies in this little habit of waking up your attention to your thoughts, actions, and feelings.

Chapter 5:

When Your Loved One Has BPD: The Road to Acceptance and Healing

It can be the most difficult feeling in the world to love someone who is suffering from a personality disorder. The rules of BPD change the relationship on any given day. It is as if you decided to play chess with a dear friend and they keep smashing the board and pieces, or even throwing them at your face.

The problem with loving someone with borderline is not that they are incapable of returning affection, trust, and intimacy. The problem is that your loved one is in a personal prison until they start getting help. It is common to feel helpless, despairing, lost, confused, or any other sort of feeling that you may not normally experience in other, more stable relationships.

The first thing to know about dealing with recovery from the effects of a relationship with a BPD is to understand that it takes time. BPD develops over the span of childhood and it takes years and sometimes decades to unravel, let alone understand. Be patient with yourself, primarily. It is a beautiful thing to be able to love another person, whether it is family or friend. It is a testament to your character that, even during some of the most challenging situations that can arise in a relationship; you still have affection for your borderline loved one.

As much as those with BPD have to relearn fundamental ways of being in relationships, those who have been raised by a BPD parent or have been in a close relationship with their patterns of behavior also have to relearn their inner sense of truth.

Ruth, a daughter of a BPD parent, grew up feeling confused about what was an appropriate feeling to have in close relationships. She recounts, "Never knowing if I was allowed to be angry, sad, or even happy at times." This is a normal experience for children of BPD parents. The disorder affects the parent's ability to maintain healthy boundaries with their children and this often leads to the parent making sure the emotional center of gravity around the house focuses on them.

Acknowledge for yourself that, even when in a love-relationship, negative feelings will arise in even the best partnerships. Those who are close to BPD individuals will have to fight harder to acknowledge the negative feelings within themselves, as the BPD parent or loved one has made a pattern to negate and invalidate these inner truths.

Acceptance

In a very personal and invisible way, reckoning with a BPD personality in your life is the classic process of grief. It is a road to acceptance marked by difficulties, steps towards acceptance, and then steps seemingly backward into denial. This is okay. Framing the experience of recovery from a borderline as a process of grief and acceptance will help you advance in the long term. If you pressure yourself to "get better" or "get over it" then you are accessing the anger and frustration you have buried about the relationship. As is common, instead of externalizing this anger and allowing it to pass through, the BPD-adjacent person will direct this anger back against themselves.

This is by design. The BPD experience will attempt to gaslight, or deny your reality, and put all blame back upon *you*. This is because a BPD individual *cannot tolerate* being wrong or feeling ashamed of their actions. Every BPD sufferer will experience this to some varying degree, but the fact that an underlying identity and sense of self is not established makes simple, honest accusations, such as, "You've hurt my feelings," go directly to the borderline's idea of self. They do not hear, "I've hurt someone," they hear, "I am intolerable to this person; I am not worthy of love." Remember the warped mental-mirror? This is the fearful translation of relationships that happen by stealth within the confines of BPD.

It may seem wise to combat these misinterpretations. It may seem as if you can *solve the problem* before it even starts. Knowledge is power, after all. As you are now educating yourself on BPD and gaining a sense of how the disorder affects and alters thinking, you may attempt to navigate this mental minefield the next time you encounter it.

Dave, a lawyer in his 60s, who has made great strides in his recovery from BPD, reflects on how his wife would try to combat his rages. "She was working treatment for her own recovery while I was doing mine, which was very helpful, I think, for certain situations. But when I was deeply triggered by an event, something as simple as her being late to pick me up from doctor's office on one occasion, I would have the overwhelming, negative anger that I was working on to accept—you know, radically," he laughs. "But, my wife knew what was going on by this point with me, and I would try to sit on my words and do the techniques DBT was teaching me to calm down. However, she would say something like, 'I know you're upset and also I did my best getting here, but there was traffic.' And it would just send me off. I'd become mean-spirited and petty. It took me a long time to understand truly the damage I was causing. I wish I could've spared her all that unnecessary hurt."

The above is a best-case scenario where there is time, effort, and a lot of hard work put into becoming more self-aware about patterns of behavior. The temptation is to think, as the loved one of someone with BPD, *I can help them! I can fix them because I know them the best! I can help make them aware of all the things they do not understand about themselves!* This is a sign of your wonderful compassion and generosity of spirit. Whenever a response like this comes up for you, take the time to acknowledge how great your capacity is for love. The hard lesson to learn, however, and those who have been in recovery for a while know that it is one of the most difficult to accept, is that BPD *is not your responsibility. Your only responsibility is to take care of yourself.*

At first, people usually blanche at this idea. *"How selfish!"* you may be thinking. The road to acceptance is the journey of recovering your own unique and independent sense of self. Too often, BPD lives are marked with the haunting sensation that they are indebted, owned by, or obligated to the BPD in their lives. This is also by design. The number one fear of the BPD individual is being abandoned. That's it. It is an intense, irrational, core fear that BPD parents and loved ones must address and overcome if they are to heal. That is not a journey you can take with them. In fact, they have most likely operated to make it feel like you *can never leave them.*

Marcy, now in her late 20s, admitted that her mom never wanted her to "leave the nest." "I felt trapped in my own home, even though I was allowed to leave, go to school, go with friends, whenever I wanted. It was just this feeling, and I have to say that it felt like a *fact*, that I just couldn't leave my mother. I felt like I could feel what she was feeling from miles away."

Personality disorders do not stop for other people's needs and desires. They are designed as a survival mechanism to protect a person who suffered such a severe trauma that they had to adopt desperate means to survive emotionally. You do not owe BPD anything. You cannot meet the core-fear of BPD. There is no way any individual can make another feel as if they will never be abandoned. It is a fact that lives change and that there is inevitable loss. The *fear of abandonment* is irrational and can never be soothed with logic, reason, or actions that prove the fear false.

If Marcy had stayed at home with her mother, rather than going off to university as she did and beginning her own life, if she had followed her mother's wishes and essentially extended her childhood indefinitely, then Marcy's mother would have still have had an enormous, endless fear of abandonment. The center of personality disorders exists almost as if they are an emotional black hole of needs. There is no way a loved one can correct this, even if it seems certain gestures of love will help. Forgoing your own personal needs to placate a person with BPD will only provide temporary relief for them and only add to further pent-up resentment for you.

Acceptance begins with removing blame. If this were easy, then the professional field of therapy would be non-existent due to its redundancy. If you know and love a person with BPD, you are most likely aware of where some of their behavior comes from. Their personal history is most likely traumatic and therefore sympathetic. It is okay to feel sympathy for their trials and tribulations. However, a rough past does not remove responsibility from present behavior.

You can accept that your BPD loved one was perhaps served a very raw deal in life while you also accept that it is not a just cause for unfair, or abusive, treatment towards you now. Try to separate these two ideas: you can have sympathy for what led to their BPD and you can also not tolerate the current terms of your relationship. This will help remove blame from your loved one having the disorder itself and help bring you into where you can hold them accountable. It is very easy to go, *"Well, they had a rough life, so I can't really fault them for anything."* In order to get anywhere in your own recovery, you must accept where fault does lie and process these emotions of disappointment, fear, and hurt.

Acceptance also needs to include the fact that *you* have experienced much grief in your relationship. This may come up for children of BPD in the sense that they lost a childhood. This is not out-of-bounds to claim. In healthy, stable households, children are raised with a sense of integrity or being able to expect consistent behavior and stability, from their parents. Children of BPD are denied this.

Carla, who was only 8 years old when she started to realize something was "off" with her mother, remembered feeling like the "weather of the house would change every day." In response, Carla would try to avoid her mother's tempers by hiding in her room and telling herself to "be a better daughter to make mom happy." No child should feel responsible for their parent's feelings. This is a role reversal of the most unjust kind when a child is expected to parent their parent. Children of BPD grow up between the extremes of being both savior and devil to their parent's moods. This is a loss of freedom, of independence, and the right to be a carefree child. It may feel quite dramatic to state to yourself, *"I lost my childhood."* Beginning to tell yourself your truth, however, is the only way to begin to heal.

Recovering Your Sense of Self

What may have been denied you in a close relationship with a BPD individual is your right to exist independently of their personality. What does this look like?

"I felt I was always being watched by my dad, even when I was living in another city. I'd go to the store, pick up a dessert, and hear his voice go, 'do not buy that.' It is hard to explain because I know other people think about their parents often, but I feel like my dad is inside of me." —Oscar, 34

"I was relieved when we finally decided to divorce because it got to the point when, at night, trying to sleep next to him, I just felt I was suffocating. I could feel his every movement in the bed as almost a silent call for my attention. I knew when he was suicidal just from the way his head hung. It was a constant marathon of worrying about him. I didn't even realize I was so angry until the divorce was final." —Mary, 42

"I just hated her so much but I couldn't stop loving her." — Lyssa, 27

BPD requires having its needs met first. If you picture a pyramid, much like Maslow's hierarchy of needs, then you know that the wider portion of the base signifies what needs the most attention. In matters of survival, this level of the pyramid is food, shelter, water, and sex. When it comes to the pyramid of a family, the base level of the pyramid should be the needs, both emotional and physical, of the children. Childhood is defined by the period of life when humans require their needs to be met by adults. Children require support, love, nurturing, food, play, exercise, and awareness that their experience is valued and validated.

This does not mean, by any stretch of the imagination, that children should run the show. For example, a three-year-old having a stress tantrum because they desperately want an ice cream but have just been told they cannot have one is a common reaction most parents are familiar with. An appropriate parenting response is to acknowledge that yes, they are upset, but they still cannot have the ice cream, and that, most importantly, they will still be okay without. The BPD parent may react in an incongruous fashion to this situation. They may begin to feel distressed by their child's cries to the point of misinterpreting the event as an indictment on their parenthood. They may believe, fully, that their child does not love them. This is then perceived as a threat of abandonment.

This is not hyperbole: the BPD parent can experience an upset from a toddler as a threat of abandonment. The reality is that, until adolescence, the only person who can abandon anyone is the parent. The BPD parent may, instead of soothing their ice-cream panicked child, attack their upset as "wrong" or "selfish" or, in extreme moments, yell about how they "wish I never had you!" It is all a dramatic play to recover a sense of security for the BPD parent. The damage, however, is that the child is confused about their own internal life. The pattern, if continued over the child's development, builds to a haunting sense that whatever they feel is wrong.

This pattern also affects adult relationships between borderline and otherwise stable personalities. Being in a close romantic relationship has a profound impact on a person's sense of well-being and perspective.

Ali, a young man who started working at a tech startup post-graduation, fell in love with his manager, a woman in her early 30s. "It was the time of my life," he said, until her BPD tendencies started to make him feel like he was completely responsible for her well-being. "I felt like, if I even looked at another girl, she would lash out. And I was just ordering coffee, you know!" His relationship lasted five years and in that time, Ali noticed a decline in his own confidence. "It was like I lost my direction, my inner direction, because all of my energy went to her. I used to be carefree and go on trips with my friends, or even know what I wanted to do with my career, but being in love with her made me start to doubt myself. I also really felt like I lost my ability to be angry. But, oh boy did that change after I got out." Ali made a point to share that he still values their time together, but for different reasons than he expected. "I think I learned a lot about myself. I didn't know that I would put up with some of the things I did, and I've worked on these areas personally since. I really loved who she is, and still do. However, I think I had to draw a line between her and what her disorder was doing to her thinking. And what it was doing to me."

Recovering from a close relationship with a BPD individual will take time and an enormous effort to relearn (or learn for the first time) how to validate your own experiences. The definition of self-esteem is only this: the ability to validate, accept, and value your inner experiences. BPD interrupts this vital sense of self in service to a core-fear that brooks no regard for other people's feelings. If you are currently feeling like you suffer from low self-esteem, do not worry. This is an aspect of the psyche that can be reborn, grown, or be strengthened with time, attention, and care. In fact, remaining curious about your life and what may be affecting it is an excellent sign that your self-esteem is in working, if albeit depressed, order. The fact you are educating yourself now on the possible difficulties of your life and how to heal them is a telltale sign of vitality. Give yourself a pat on the back right now for finding extraordinary ways to persist and survive within the harrowing chambers of BPD.

Ask yourself a few questions now to gain a sense of how BPD has affected you:

- When met with a conflict at work, school, or home, how certain do I feel about myself that I can constructively manage the situation? Do I fear retaliation or saying the wrong thing?
- Do I tend to avoid looking to others for help or a reality-check about my life and goals? If so, what feelings prevent me from considering other people's views?
- Am I able to accept criticism and decide if it truly applies to me? Do I avoid any situation that may lead to criticism?
- Is it true when I'm making plans, I feel confident about my decisions? Or, do I always have a sense that it should've been a different choice after I've made a commitment?
- Do my relationships bring me a sense of contentment and validation? Or do my relationships, whether with family or friends, bring me a sense of insecurity and unease?

A strong sense of self can manage the wear-and-tear of other people's opinions, criticism, and confrontation. A victim of BPD and those surrounding its wake will have difficulties standing up for themselves (which is not surprising, as it is directly a missing "self" which is at stake). If you suspect you are grappling with issues of self-worth, self-validation, emotional fluidity (being able to feel a wide range of emotions), or general lack of self-esteem, then professional guidance would be more than appropriate to help navigate your journey.

Self-help reading is fantastic and can support your efforts in a more fulfilling sense of self. The irony is that self-help is most effective with a strong and clear sense of self. Talking to a licensed therapist is a good place to start. Even if your loved one has not yet obtained an official diagnosis of BPD, or may for various reasons and limitations (either personal or circumstantial) never obtain an official diagnosis, an educated counselor trained in BPD can help you manage the impact it has had on your life.

Chapter 6:

Day-to-Day Techniques for Self-Improvement

You now have a general overview of Borderline Personality Disorder. This chapter will give you actionable tools you can start using now to better your circumstance, whether you have BPD, or are supporting a loved one with the diagnosis. As stated before, BPD is a clinical diagnosis, not a judgment. This book, nor others, can serve as an official diagnosis or treatment. The advice offered here is for personal benefit and should be only used in conjunction with proper care.

Most of the advice here will apply to both those diagnoses and those who have loved ones with BPD. This does not mean that those who are close to BPD also have, or "catch," the disorder. The model for recovery efforts for BPD shares a similar structure to Alcoholics Anonymous and Al-Anon. The former group focuses on the twelves steps as they relate to their addiction. Al-Anon, a support group for those who have had close relationships or been affected by another person's alcoholism, also works the same steps, but through a filter of their specific relationship to alcoholism and loving someone who is suffering. The steps remain the same because, just as with managing BPD, the necessary tools remain unchanged: self-awareness, self-soothing, and therapeutic work.

Encouraging Self-Awareness: Identifying Negative Patterns of Thought

Understanding negative patterns of thought can be liberating, especially to those who have never felt able to control negative self-image and feelings of low self-worth. Those who suffer from BPD will have definitely experienced at least one out of the following list of negative thinking distortions. Those who live close to the disorder will perhaps adopt or be encouraged to repeat these thinking patterns to match a warped reality as well. A brief introduction of each cognitive distortion follows as it applies to BPD, as well as an exercise to encourage self-awareness of these harbingers of negative self-thought.

Polarized Thinking is the classic borderline pattern of all-or-nothing thinking. Either someone is perfect and good, or they are unworthy and a failure. There is no in between. If a conversation is going well, then it is okay, but if there is one small deviation from comfortable feelings between its participants, it is a disaster. Getting a new job after applying to it means that you are a success, but if it falls through, then there is nothing good coming your way, ever.

The hallmark of this pattern of thinking is vocabulary words like "always," "never," and "total." In this kind of thinking-world, the stakes are always too high and the disappointments all too debilitating to the self. In actuality, nothing and no one is "perfect" or "a total success." Life holds shades of grey for everyone and this is not limiting, but freeing. Pay attention to your thoughts after a perceived triumph or disappointment. How do you talk to yourself? Does it make you anxious about being too hopeful or too full of despair? What is actually the truth in the situation?

Catastrophizing easily appears in the mind of BPD. Watching television news and hearing a sad report of a car accident engenders a thought pattern of, *"What if it was I? It will happen to me! Oh my goodness, what about so and so, no one should drive cars anymore!"* Making a catastrophe out of the events of life serves no one any good.

In the rare event of an actual catastrophe, there are still ways in which to isolate the event from staining the possibility of other events also turning into a disaster. When you begin to feel untethered by bad news, or a paranoia about a distressing event rises out of nowhere, ask yourself, *"Am I blowing things out of proportion? What likelihood is there really of this disaster happening? Did the likelihood increase within the minute that I just began to think about it? What inspired me to start thinking this way?"*

Catastrophizing also stretches in the positive, aggrandizing direction. Catastrophizing thoughts might have you thinking that someone else's qualities make them perfect, or their recent successes are so many miles above your own. This sort of distorted thinking can also minimize events that should be held with value and importance. For example, minimizing your personal achievements and qualities can be a way to self-catastrophize. The thinking may also be used to ignore red flags in a relationship and to downplay how significant someone else's imperfections are. You can start by asking if what you are thinking and feeling about yourself or another person is appropriate. You can also check to see if the opposite seems true. If you believe an event to be a mistake that qualifies as a "disaster," can you check and see if you think anyone else sees it the same way? Just ask internally. Begin to acknowledge that there are many ways to look at a situation before feeling that your experience is the conclusive truth of it.

Personalization is a favorite of the BPD disposition. This thinking is a distortion that has a person believe that other's actions and feelings are a direct response to their own behavior or thinking. The truth is that people exist independent of our lives and our thoughts. If you walk into a room and people look up and seem bored, it is not because *you* are boring them.

Personalization makes these moments seem to have a direct origin from the distorted thinker.

This thought pattern also leads people to take responsibility for events they had nothing to do with. A BPD woman may take responsibility for a natural disaster that happened on the other side of the world. "If only I had been a better person!" she would cry in response for an explanation. This may seem extreme, but distorted thinking does not stop for logic. The *feeling* of it is true for the BPD individual and that feeling is as good as proof. Try to separate personalization thoughts from the truth that everyone has a unique experience on this planet.

You may start to recognize this kind of thinking and remind yourself, "I felt very uncomfortable and also I cannot know what that other person was actually thinking. He looked uncomfortable and that does not mean I made him uncomfortable." It is hopefully a relief to remind yourself you are not responsible for every event in the world! The compassionate reality is this thinking is a way of taking control of a world that was once very much out of control. It is a noble attempt to make sense of the often-illogical course of events and emotions in life, but personalization ends up only hurting the self by attaching too much guilt to non-events.

Do you readily blame yourself for the action of others? Do you see bad events and try to understand how you may have caused them? Is it difficult for you to step back and not be involved in other people's upsets and crises? If so, beware of the role personalization may have within your thought patterns.

Control Fallacies are distorted thoughts that lead one to believe they are under someone else's control, not their own. There are two breeds of this distorted thinking: external and internal control. While external control fallacies are less common for the borderline individual, its mark can be apparent in situations where accountability is offloaded onto another. For example, a project deadline is not met not because of the BPD individual's behavior, but *because my children distracted me too much.* Internal control fallacies appear as taking responsibility for everyone's emotional states. *My partner is upset and it must be my fault.* Direction, internal, or external, either gives a false sense of control or being controlled and will either inundate or obfuscate responsibility in personal interactions.

Jumping to Conclusions applies to both people and events. This distorted pattern will make it seem possible to read the motivations and feeling states of others without having confirmation these readings are correct. "I know she's mad at me because I know!" a borderline individual might declare without room for the fact that, without asking, there is no way to know why someone is upset. This also applies to forecasting the future and assuming events will turn out positively or negatively without a balanced view of the possibility. In both cases, distorted thoughts that jump to conclusions evade the discomfort and uncertainty of *not knowing.* BPD individuals will habitually jump to conclusions to avoid this uncertainty. If things are uncertain, that means things can rapidly change. It is easier for the borderline to jump to an even negative conclusion rather than tolerate the uncertainty of a relationship or something possibly ending poorly.

Filtering is the selective process of only focuses on the negative implications in a situation and removing all the positives. Jenny goes to a party and feels very shy. Her goal is to talk to a few new people and hopefully meet a nice looking boy. She spends the evening having a laugh with her friends and does end up meeting a few new people but does not connect with any potential dates. Instead of being proud of overcoming her shyness and having a good time, Jenny focuses on thoughts that tell her the party was a complete failure and that, since no attractive boys ended up chatting with her, she is unlovable. She spends the next week focusing on how she chose the wrong dress to wear and how she probably scared people off with her "too loud" laugh. This can go on and on when nothing from reality supports Jenny's thinking.

BPD loves filtering events because it helps support the inner chaos and turmoil that feeds the disorder. If borderlines fear being abandoned, then a constant mental tape of details that focus on how inevitable being alone and abandoned will help trick the borderline individual into believing the worst-case scenario will come true. This creates a reality where all of BPD's distinctive behaviors still make sense. Filtering thoughts is just like the Instagram concept of using filters to make reality look better, except in this case, the filter paints a picture of how grim reality feels for the borderline individual.

Overgeneralization is a form of distorted thinking that turns one event into a rule for all time. BPD individuals will often rush to overgeneralize as a matter of self-defense. While missing the bus and running late for work one day is irritating, the borderline man may then tell himself that he's always late for work and he is a lost cause. This prevents him from seeing the hectic day as a one-time event and serves to protect himself from taking responsibility for getting to work on time. He may get to the office and, when asked why he was behind, respond in a dramatic, "Well, I'm just a waste who can't get anywhere on time." This is an overgeneralization and counterintuitively protects an individual from facing the consequences of an action or event. Pay attention to any broad themes you may ascribe to yourself in life. Do you feel you are always losing things? Always lost? Certain to never succeed? Certain to never be loved? Why do you think this is inevitable? What evidence is there to support your case? Did one bad experience color your entire future? Is this fair?

The Fallacy of Fairness is a delicate thought distortion that is very individual. The idea of fairness can make living in the world extremely inhospitable. The fallacy of fairness takes a situation and turns it into an internal weapon. A friend may have recently announced her engagement and she spreads the word on social media. Her BPD friend sees this as an injustice, as she is the one who has been single for longer, and the world should couple those who have been waiting the longest. Now, this assessment would be very specific to the BPD friend's sense of justice and may sound absurd to another. This is why it is important to note when a sense of righteousness enters your thoughts. What do you think is unfair in life? When do you turn that sense of unfairness inwards, and hold resentment about "unfair" treatment? Are there other ways of looking at the situation as neither fair nor unfair, but just a fact of life?

Blaming is a frequently used distortion of borderline personalities. Blame means placing responsibility where it should not go. Blame can look like making someone else responsible for our feelings. *You make me so jealous!* The fallacy here is that no one can make you feel anything. Your emotions are part of your private domain. Yes, people act and say things that cause you to react.

However, as impossible as it may sound, you choose your emotions. That's right! If anything, the most honest statement you can make in a distressing situation is, *"You have said very insulting things to me and I'm allowing you to make me feel enraged."* That is an apt description of what is going on. Although everyone, not just BPD or other personality disorders, struggles with this actuality. Ask yourself honestly if you believe you can choose your emotions. If not, who chooses how to make you feel? If that person no longer existed, who would then determine how you feel? Can you change how you feel when you're alone? When you're in a group? If so, how do you start to change? What in your life would change if you were responsible for how you felt in any situation?

Emotional Reasoning is the difficulty to separate feeling from fact. *I feel ugly so I am ugly.* Staying in the realm of feelings as facts is a dizzying, unrewarding venture. Feelings must remain distinct from evidence and reality. A famous Radiohead lyric goes: *Just 'cause you feel it / Doesn't mean it's there.* BPD creates a world where feelings are prioritized over reality. Save yourself from the changeable nature of an emotional-fueled definition of life by spotting when emotional reasoning comes into play. What do you believe is true because it feels true? If you feel like a failure, does that honestly mean you'll never succeed at a goal in life?

Shoulds are distorted thoughts that focus on rigid rules for life. They are often used to punish the self. *I should start running three times a week, I should do the dishes, I should call my mother more.* What sneaks in under the radar is the idea that you are breaking the rules by not follow strict self-orders. Anytime you tell yourself "should" you are setting yourself up for guilt.

BPD individuals will lock themselves up in a cage of shoulds in order to punish themselves for "being bad." What happens when you don't get up at the hour you "should" get up at? A barrage of self-criticism that can spiral into a negative outlook for the whole day. A more constructive approach is to focus on the empowering reason behind the commitment or choice. *I want to have more endurance so I would like to run three times a week, I feel more peaceful when the dishes are finished so I'll do that before bed, I like when my mom says she feels*

71

better after I call so I will call her more. This brings warmth, encouragement, and self-love into decision-making rather than authoritarian commands.

How often do you tell yourself you "should" do something? Pick one of these shoulds right now and think about why you want to do the task. Can you reframe the goal in terms of how you'll benefit from its achievement?

Always Being Right is a cognitive distortion that flares up when an individual experiences being "wrong" about something as being "wrong" within themselves. This distorted thought pattern would attack perceived opponents in order to win an argument *at any cost*. This includes the loss of friendship or hurt feelings. One may think it's a sense of pride that encourages this thinking pattern, but it is actually a lack of self-esteem. Those with a solid sense of self-respect can allow for disagreements, as these differences have no effect on who that person is.

BPD individuals do not have this baseline of self-esteem. They perceive themselves to be whatever is going on emotionally for them at the moment. If they are "wrong" in an argument, then they *are wrong* and feel ashamed. This is avoided through stubborn, winner-takes-all arguments. Do you feel a need to be right all the time? When you are wrong or make a mistake, can you own up to it easily? What would happen if you said you were in error? How would you feel?

Heaven's Reward Fallacy is the myth that there is a morality scoreboard that keeps track of sacrifices and self-denials and will reward those who play the martyr. When these restrictive practices are not rewarded then resentment builds. Those close to a BPD loved one may fall into this distorted thinking pattern, as it is easy for victims of borderline behavior to learn to negate their wants and needs. This can be internalized as a play to gain later reward from their BPD loved one. A child who begins to see that their parent prefers their silence at home might be quiet for an entire weekend, hoping to receive their parent's praise. When it does not come, then their heart is broken.

Who benefits from you suffering? What do you expect when you make sacrifices for someone else? If you do not receive thanks for your time or energy, do you become angry or resentful? While there is a human need for appreciation and thanks, working to shift the heaven's reward fallacy into something less covert is healthy. No one should suffer in silence under the expectation it will guarantee a reward.

The Counterbalance to Negative Thought Patterns: Affirmations

After becoming familiar with the above-disordered thinking patterns, you have probably come across a few that feel close to home. These thought patterns are not unique to BPD and everyone has, to some degree, these habitual ways of coping with stressful or unexpected situations. The first step is to learn how to recognize and categorize a negative thought when it occurs.

Do not worry about being 100% accurate about which category the thought falls into. If you are waiting in line at the grocery checkout and a toddler starts having a hissy fit in front of you, you may be rightly annoyed. Perhaps your feeling of annoyance turns into thoughts of *I hate being around children, I always get annoyed with children, children probably hate me, even when I was a kid, no one liked me...* This series of instantaneous, unconscious thinking has several distorted patterns within it. There is overgeneralization of "all children hating me," filtering of focusing on the child in the grocery checkout and no other details about the day, personalization that the child crying has anything to do with you, and the emotional reasoning that, since you feel like children hate you, they obviously do. None of this is true! However, it comes up quick and fast and will change your mood in a minute.

It is not so important to capture and identify each distorted thought pattern. What is important is to begin to detach from their power. To do this, you need to be armed with affirmations. Affirmations are planned, positive statements that are in place to respond to decided events. The most useful affirmations affirm your reality while including others. For example, it makes no sense to tell yourself, "I am happy," when you are upset. Affirmations are not about lying to yourself. The only way to build real self-esteem is to tell yourself the truth.

The truth, however, includes the wider world, which is sometimes hazy or even mystifying for the borderline personality. A better affirmation is, when upset, "I am upset, and it is not the end of the world. People are upset all the time and it passes." Finding a few clear, simple, and direct affirmations can work wonders when any of the distorted patterns of thought come into play. Review the list of suggested affirmations for difficult situations below and see if any click for you. If so, take out a note and jot the affirmation down. Place this note somewhere visible, such as your nightstand or on your fridge, as a reminder that you can always access the words whenever you need. To encourage your use of affirmations, after reading the below list, write five of your own empowering affirmations. Remember, the key is to affirm your worldview and the fact that there are other possibilities outside of your own.

Affirmations for Anger

I am angry and I have had this feeling before. I will survive.

Just because I am angry does not mean I need to take it out on anyone.

I love myself just as I am, even when angry. I love other people, even when they have anger.

Anger is upsetting and it upsets other people, too. I am not alone.

Affirmations for Sadness

I have sadness right now. That does not make me a sad person. What is true now does not mean it will always be true.

I give myself time to be sad. I love myself enough to give myself that space.

What he said is upsetting me. Right now, I am sad about it. I may feel differently later.

It is no one's fault that I am sad. It is not my fault and it is not my family's fault. Emotions always come and go.

Affirmations for Jealousy

Her success means that success is possible. I celebrate the success of others because I want them to celebrate my own.

Jealousy feels awful and I will let it pass. People feel jealousy every day.

I notice that jealousy leads me to feel impatient with myself. I give myself time to feel what I need to. There is no rush.

Your turn. Go ahead and write five affirmations that speak to you. They can be very general and gentle or very straightforward. Whatever makes you feel more in control and settled in yourself is good. Refer back to Chapter 4's emotional bank account exercise to review distressing moments when a strong affirmation may have been useful. You can use these self-inventories for inspiration.

The secret is that all affirmations, no matter how they're phrased, share a common message. That message is that you are strong, capable, and willing to change for the better. What better message is that?

Further Readings

Understanding BPD is a life-long journey and there is much to explore. One of the best ways to learn about the disorder for yourself or loved ones is to continue your reading on the subject. Your therapist or psychologist will have a recommendation list as well, and they will be very open to discussing your thoughts and reactions as you absorb the growing literature on the subject. The following titles are becoming touchstones for those looking for answers to this complex personality disorder. A list of highly recommended reading follows:

I Hate You—Don't Leave Me: Understanding the Borderline Personality by Jerold J. Kreisman and Hal Straus

Stop Walking on Eggshells (2nd Edition) by Paul T. Mason, MS and Randi Kreger

Surviving a Borderline Parent: How to Heal Your Childhood Wounds & Build Trust, Boundaries, and Self-Esteem by Kimberlee Roth and Freda B. Friedman, Ph.D., LCSW

The Borderline Personality Disorder Survival Guide: Everything You Need to Know About Living with BPD by Alexander L. Chapman, Ph.D. and Kim L. Gratz, Ph.D.

The Dialectical Behavior Therapy Skills Workbook: Practical DBT Exercises for Learning Mindfulness, Interpersonal Effectiveness, Emotion Regulation, and Distress Tolerance by Matthew McKay Ph.D., Jeffrey C. Wood PsyD, and Jeffrey Brantley MD

Conclusion

Thanks for making it through to the end of *Unlocking the Mystery of Borderline Personality Disorder: A Survival Guide to Living and Coping with BPD for You and Your Loved Ones.* Let's hope it was informative and able to provide you with all of the tools you need to achieve your goals whatever they may be.

The next step is to reflect. Whether after reading you now see your own mental health in a different light, or you see someone you love struggling with Borderline Personality Disorder (BPD) tendencies, the most important message you can take home is that it is not your fault.

The origins of BPD are complex, not linear, and span over decades of development. BPD is a maladaptive response to trauma that expresses itself as a severe fear of abandonment. This fear is real and not imaginary. However, the event that led to this fear is now over and it is time to begin to let it go and heal.

The often self-destructive patterns of behavior were created by BPDs for the noble purpose of survival. Overall, a BPD is a person who is trying to survive a trauma that is long in the past, but its power still resides in the present. This is why it can be so confusing, disheartening, frightening, and a host of valid responses for those who love someone with BPD.

There are many resources for both parties to find strength and heal. A necessary step is finding appropriate, informed professional support, especially with a practitioner who specializes in Dialectical Behavior Therapy (DBT), a cognitive therapy developed to treat Borderline behavior. DBT has improved the lives of many of those living with BPD.

Participation in treatment combats one of the most difficult obstacles in healing BPD: denial. By reading this book and becoming more informed, you have already improved your situation as it shows a willingness to understand. Practice as much compassion and acceptance for yourself as you can. You are doing your best, one day at a time.

Finally, if you found this book useful in any way, a review on Amazon is always appreciated! Thank you!

Made in the USA
Monee, IL
08 May 2020